I0486137

SUICIDAL BEHAVIOR

LEARN HOW TO RECOGNIZE SUICIDAL BEHAVIOR IN YOUR FRIENDS AND FAMILY

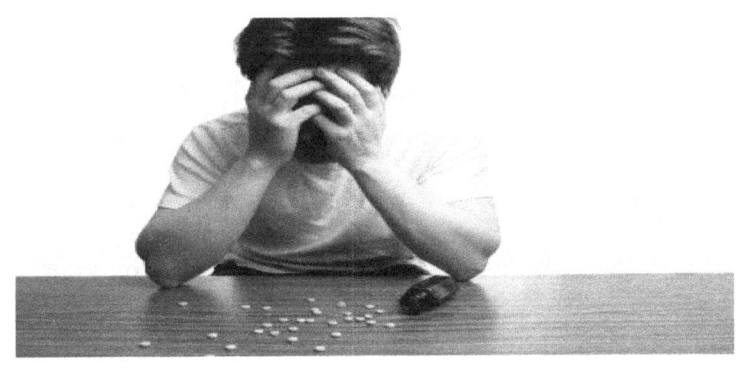

By Patricia A Carlisle

Introduction

I want to thank you and congratulate you for choosing the book, *"SUICIDE BEHAVIOR: Learn How to Recognize Suicidal Behavior In Your Friends And Family"*.

This book contains proven steps and strategies on how to recognize suicidal behavior in your friends and family.

Suicidal acts and attempts are phenomena that have been committed from one generation to another all around the world. Why do some people attempt suicide? There are various reasons that may warrant such a thing. Perhaps the most populous and famous suicide committed in the history of mankind was the one carried out by JUDAS ISCARIOT.

Judas Iscariot betrayed Jesus Christ of Nazareth according to the Christian Bible, and the motive behind it was a greed for money. He betrayed his master when he was given some pieces of silver to aid the scribes to capture Jesus, since he (Jesus) was very elusive. There are also many instances other than financial or materials rewards that warrants an individual to commit suicide.

But before we go on, let us define the term suicide and suicidal behavior. Hence, suicide is the act, or an instance of taking one's own life voluntarily, or intentionally especially when this is done by a person of a sane and sound mind. For any person to be said to have committed suicide, the person must have carried out the act without external assistance, or external intervention, or receiving help from a third party. It must be free from any person's compulsion. It must be done by a single individual, and when this happens then it is crystal clear that the case is suicidal.

Thanks again for choosing this book, I hope you enjoy it!

ABOUT THE AUTHOR

Patricia A. Carlisle, MSW, CBT

Patricia Carlisle- a Cognitive Behavioral Therapist (CBT) gives out an expression of how important it is for an individual to take into consideration the concept of self-assessment to know what human, technical and conceptual skills they posses to perform or to achieve what they desire, or to deal with everyday life. However, every particular group of people has their own unique set of ideas, traditions and events including the frame of mind according to which people perform but there are many who faces problems and fail to maintain a healthy mind set affecting their behaviors and performance to those around them.

People like Patricia Carlisle are among those who have felt this urge of serving people and helping them out of their mental crisis towards a healthy life. She has experienced some close encounters in her personal life regarding mental health issues in her family and friends that has encouraged her to pursue this as her career.

Currently Patricia Carlisle is serving as a Certified On-Line Cognitive Behavioral Therapist with an extensive 15years of experience using Cognitive-Behavior Therapy Techniques. She envisions a world where everyone gets mental health treatment with no mental health stigma and to make it real she has already set up her own Holistic Measure Online Comprehensive Behavioral Healthcare Company after retiring from The Nord Center in The Partial Hospitalization Program (PHP) Dept for 5 years and Murtis H. Taylor Mental Health Center as a mental health counselor, psychological support technician and case manager for 10 years to emulsify her skills more professionally. Along with this, she has wrote down her passion as a clinician in 25 or more short books to help individuals and families get their life back, freeing them of the restraints of negative thinking, anxiety and depression by using different approaches. She is highly appreciated among her clients for her flexibility and professionalism of dealing with them graciously.

To reach her, make use of her direct website address: http://therapist2013.wix.com/e-therapy . As she is ready to inspire hope and contribute to health and well-being by providing the best online health care through comprehensive practice, education and research.

TABLE OF CONTENT

Chapter 1

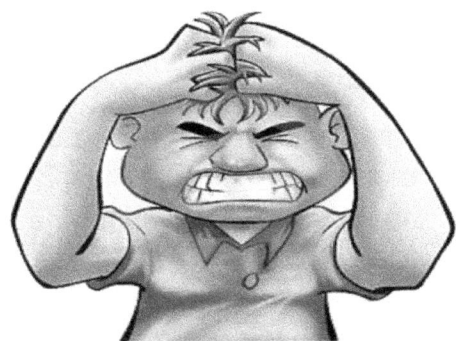

WHAT IS SUICIDAL BEHAVIOR

Suicidal behavior is when a single individual begins to exhibit certain eccentric characteristics that is suspicious, or even contrary to normal day to day life behavior which appears to be strange, and having the inclination of having the ambition, or nursing a mindset that will prompt or make the individuals to commit suicide very soon, or in the nearest future. It shows that the idea was premeditated and planned by the individual to carry out the act, and may not necessary be an accident.

There are many reasons why people attempt suicide, as discussed in the first paragraph (i.e the issue of Judas Iscariot), his own case was that of greed and love for money. He was the person in charge of keeping money for the disciples of our Lord Jesus Christ, and the bible says "he was a pilferer, that he formed the habit of stealing from the treasury, and when the option of pieces of silver was presented to him, he couldn't resist it, and he because of the assisted in the arrest of Jesus Christ when he betrayed his master with a Kiss. Probably, he thought that his master will somehow escape, but everyone knew what he had done. He couldn't bear the shame and stigma, and instead of him to seek for forgiveness he went and committed suicide.

Now what can we draw from the popular example above? We can see how..

(1) greed for money led to a betrayal.

(2) Judas was despair, hopeless, felt miserable about what he had done, and it dawn on him that he had acted adversely to the expectation or the right standard of a normal human being.

(3) He knew that his master was a righteous, just an innocent man who did not deserve to be arrested by the scribes and Pharisee, and put to death eventually.

We also have instances when people commit suicide, or attempt to commit suicide when they are suffering from depression. Some of the attempted suicides always think their situation is hopeless, and they are being frustrated by their problems, they find it so difficult to cope, or live further with it in life. They may probably think that they cannot bear their problems any longer, and that is the reasons to resort to taking their lives as the last resort.

Chapter 2

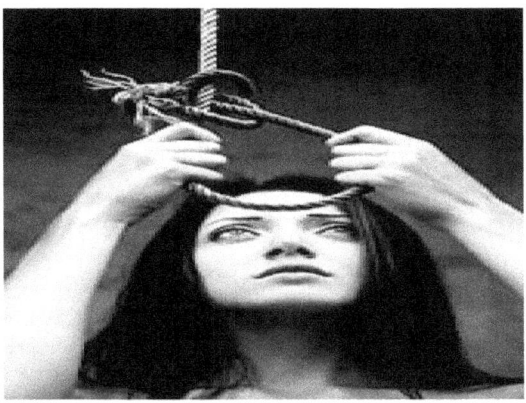

WAYS SUICIDE IS COMMENTED

Some commit suicide when they have a breakup in their relationship, when they are being cheated and abandoned by the person whom they love so much, and as we all know love is very strong. Someone may take his or her life because of a jilted lover.

Another category which appears to be more of an uprising and modern is "suicide bombing". This monster is one of the most deadliest and dreadful kind of suicidal behavior ever witness since the time of creation, because not only does the suicide bomber kills him or herself, but they drag other people around the scene of the bombing into death. Many of the suicide bombers usually have reasons for carrying out the act. The first on the list of reasons why they attempt suicide bombing is religious believes and hatred. It is very common among the religious extremist who believe that they are fighting a just cause for God. They also have this erroneous believe that there is a reward for carrying out the suicide bombing, and it is eternal life in paradise, and marriage to several virgins.

How unfortunate this is! Many countries have been dealt a fetal blow by the activities of suicide bombers who have also become terrorists by killing themselves, and also killing many people along with them. Countries in the Middle East, Asian continent, Africa, and some part of Europe and America, have also fallen victims of the activities of suicide bombers. The September 11 attack on the twin Tower building in America is one example of a devastating suicide bombing by terrorist who hijacked two passenger aircraft to carry out the dastardly act.

Over 18,000 people have lost their lives recently in a North East Africa, North West of Cameroun, Niger and Chad as a result of the immoral activities of terrorist, and suicide bombers. The African countries have been held siege for almost a decade; they weren't prepared, and were also not familiar with the trend.

Chapter 3

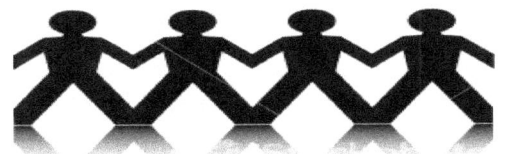 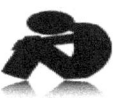

HOW TO RECOGNIZE SUICIDAL BEHAVIOR IN YOUR FRIENDS AND FAMILY

According to studies made so far, suicidal behavior comes in different facets, it could be self developed, caused by depression, disorders, stress disorders, post traumatic stress disorders, schizophrenia, anxiety disorders, and the more recent one is the indoctrination by terrorist through religious extremism given to suicide bombers. So many times the suicide person may not be suffering from any mental illness, but they are conscious of what they are doing, and knows completely that he or she is going to die in the process.

How then can you determine when someone close to you has suicidal behavior?

Moodiness: The most common thing is when the person appears to be moody, when we talk about moodiness here; we are referring to a type of moodiness that appears to take a very long time to disappear you will likely observe in the person mood swings, unexpected rage, and sudden change in normal manner of conversation. When these signs begin to emerge which is little bit unlike the person's character, then you can begin to suspect suicidal behavior.

Despair: Suicide attempted persons always feel despair about their situations, they generally have future uncertainty, and feel no hope for a better future. This is further married when the situation becomes so bad when the person is either jobless, or feels lonely and always found living a solitude life. If you notice this phenomena in someone be concerned about the welfare of such person to curtail the suicide attempts.

Nightmares: Some of the suicide attempts do normally have nightmares, or premonition of their impending death. Many times these occurrences are not properly managed. Instead of sharing the problems, the suicide attempters often become afraid, or even if they share it, it will take a psychologically gifted person to actually draw references from the experiences of the victim. That is why if this person does not get the requisite counseling and therapy, the probability of a suicide attempt is very possible. Some of them do always talk about their impending death, they may not know the form in which it will come, but if it is premeditated then they are just waiting for the time that they actually want to take their live.

Unprecedented quietness: If you notice one who has been undergoing depression for a very long time. And suddenly the mood changes, and there is a steadfast quietness and silence, then this kind of indication is dangerous, once a person remains calm unexpectedly, that means there is something going on, and it has reached a climax, a plan is about to be executed, and the victim is silence and thinking how he or she is going to slip away, either they decides to take a poison, such is common to silent suicide attempters.

A withdrawn Lifestyle: When it is noticeable that a person suddenly becomes an introvert, no longer feels comfortable to mingle and socialize with people. It is obvious also in the person's situation that nothing ever excites him or her any longer. When others are laughing they don't laugh, when people around them crack jokes, it does not appear funny to them. Most of the time the person appears to be absent minded, totally oblivion on the happenings in his environment, and many times he or she does not bat their eyelid even when they are in a noisy environment. What goes on in the mind of this person can be none other than depression that has gone nearer to a suicide point. He or she is just waiting to perpetrate the act.

Behavioral Changes: A suicide person is bound to change his or her behavior either for bad, or the way they dress may become so alien to what they usually puts on. They may become blind to what they are wearing, and do not care about what people think about their new lifestyle. If you notice a change in behavior as explained here, try to put the person under surveillance, you will see that the person will have a particular spot he or she likes to sit and meditate on something that they is harboring in their mind. That is one of the behavioral traits of a person contemplating a suicide attempt.

Taking expensive Risk: One of the ways to identify someone who is capable of committing suicide is when you notice such person is a risk taker, and do not care about the consequences of his or her actions. Dangerous acts of reckless driving, out of control, and taking over dozes of deadly drugs, excessive alcohol consumption, and acts that tend to shorten the life of the individual is an indication that the person's behavior is suicidal. You might be travelling on a train, and you see someone attempting to climb on the train, jumping out of a moving vehicle, standing in front of a fast moving vehicle etc. these are suicidal behavioral characteristics.

Some life experiences: Certainly there are some unfortunate life experiences that may tend to prompt or trigger up suicide attempt, such as loss of job, break up in a relationship, loss of a loved one, losing a championship or title, under-achievements, severe illness like terminal disease, financial crises and poverty are some of the events in a man's life that can cause him to commit suicide.

Making Arrangements: If you notice that someone is making arrangements for something, and in the process he or she plans to give out some of their properties to people around him; he or she decides to make a WILL in the process, he or she further makes visits to their friends or relation, you can begin to suspect them of a possible suicide attempt. Most arranged, premeditated and planned suicide attempters often leave a notice behind on the table while they hanged themselves in their room, or by drinking poison. On the note, they are always sincere with the reasons for committing suicide. It has always been the case, either the person leaves a note, or he or she leaves a video footage behind to show why they committed suicide.

Suicide Threat: If you listen to conversation from people within and around you, and you happen to hear someone say something like **"you leave me, I'm going to commit suicide"**, or you see a daughter telling her father **"I'm going to marry him, and if you try to stop me I'll commit suicide"**. Perhaps not all these cases always result to attempting suicide, however, all suicide threats should always be taken seriously, to make sure to save that person from the supposed attempt.

When the person No longer Values Life: A suicide person will no longer value the worthiness of life, he or she will always at some point say words like **"life is not worth**

living", when you hear such words from a person, know that that person is showing that behavioral tendencies of committing suicide.

When you hear someone tell one of the family members that "**they are better off when he or she is not around them**" that means the person is thinking something, don't be surprise, he or she may stun the entire family by committing suicide.

Dangerous weapon: When the person acquires a dangerous weapon, the first thing that should come to mind is, what does this person need a weapon for? Is either he or she going to use it on somebody, or they are going to one day use it on them self.

Possession of Poisonous substances: The person may even be found with poisonous substances, and when you ask the person what he or she wants to use it for, and they lie about it, or is not giving you a genuine reason, know that they may likely commit suicide, for instance, a person is not having a farm, but he purchases a chemical meant to be used on plants or crops, brings it into the house in the city, or brings in some other chemicals known to be poisonous into the house.

Statements like "**next time I will take enough pills to get the job done**", when a person makes this kind of statement, be weary of such person. It means the first attempt at suicide made was situation when someone makes voluntary statements like "**never mind or don't worry, I will not be around to deal with the situation as it pleases you**". This kind of statement is a clear indication that the person is up to something, and they will likely commit suicide, or is proposing to attempt one.

Another instance is when somebody makes a derogatory statement like "**you will be sorry when I am gone**" this is another situation where suicide attempts can be deduced from the statements of an individual who is contemplating suicide. This is one of the most implicating statements that are very common among people who are prone to suicidal behavior. Immediately you notice such statements, you can suspect that this person has a suicidal behavior, and may tend to commit it sooner or later. Also when the person makes such statement like "**I will not come your way any longer or any further**", this is another statement that can suggest to you to assume suicidal behavior.

When there is a perception about the difficulty of life, and the person always shows remorse, and regrets about life, and says he or she can no longer cope with the hard times. Sometimes such individual begin to gradually withdraw from the public, and tend to live a solitude life where it will finally lead them to commit suicide. Also, when the person makes mention of averments like "**I will not be a burden to you any longer**", most especially when the person has been suffering from a disease (either terminal or not), you will always get to hear such words, this person always feels you have done so much for him or her, and probably being alive constitutes a burden on you, and may decide to take his or her life as an option to relieve you of all you efforts at taking care of them.

Another typical example is when somebody says words like "**Why is it that nobody understands me**?", or "**that nobody cares about them**", or "**that nobody feels the way I do**", often these categories of people who suffer this kind of psychological syndrome may end up being confused as to why things are really the way they are, they always feel disappointed, and when this happens suicidal behavior begins to build gradually until it reaches a climax where the individual is capable of taking his own life.

Some suicidal behavior is traceable to people who think that **"there is nothing they can do to make things better in life"**, when disappointments sets in, they will always contemplate suicide when the problems they are facing becomes unbearable. Some will always make dangerous suggestions like **"I'm better off when I am dead"**, to them they believe that not being alive, or being dead is the best thing for them to have a peace of mind. Also when a person **"has the feeling that there is no way out of a problem or impending doom"**, the individual may decide to commit suicide out-rightly. Some warlords who happened to have suffered a lost in the battle field for instance, always decide to take their lives instead of surrendering to their enemies. So, when it comes to a point that a person feels there is no way out, he may decide to commit suicide, when you see somebody say words like **'there is no way out'** in a situation, the person is showing suicidal behavior.

Suicidal behavior is traceable to someone who does not care about the feelings of others, about him, or about other people's survival, when they depend on him. When someone says words like **"you will be better off when I am not around"** then if he goes off to commit suicide, don't be surprised, because to them they have already delivered the message, such behavior is suicidal.

Conclusion

Thank you again for choosing this book!

I hope this book was able to help you to identify suicidal behavior.

The wave of suicide attempts around the world is alarming, it cuts across every continent, one thing is certain, and that is "most suicide attempts are contemplated', and before the person commits suicide there are some inherent changes in behavior that the person will exhibit before he or she commits the act, most common among these behavior are depression, despair, hopelessness, and so many possible frustration caused by circumstances that can lead to the commission of suicide.

Hence, suicidal behavior is something that has to do with situations that leads to the commission of the act caused by what an individual experiences in his surrounding environment that prompts a change in a person's normal behavior, and showing inclinations towards behavior that is suicidal.

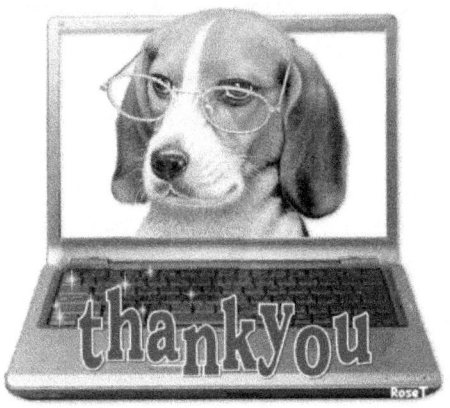

Finally, if you enjoyed this book, would you be kind enough to leave a review for this book on Amazon? It'd be greatly appreciated!

Click here to leave a review for this book on Amazon!

Thank you and good luck!

Preview Of 'UNDERSTANDING SUICIDE'

Chapter 1

SUICIDE THROUGH HISTORY

Every year approximately 30,000 people die by suicide in the United States, and one million worldwide. Approximately 650,000 people yearly receive emergency treatment after attempting suicide in the United States. It is the third leading course of death among American youths and the eleventh for Americans of all ages. Over the last 100 years suicides have out-numbered homicides by at least 3 to 2. Almost 4 times as many Americans died by suicide than in the Vietnam War during the same time period.

The rates of suicide are exceptionally high among certain populations; white males over 75 years of age, Native Americans, and certain profession(e.g., health professions, police). The rates among youth are rising. For decades, the federal government of the United States has been concerned about high suicide rates. Thirty years after the first national effort was established at the National Institute of Mental Health in 1969, the Surgeon General of the United States issued a "Call to Action to Prevent Suicide." Soon after, a National Strategy for Suicide Prevention (2001) presented a comprehensive assessment of future goals and objectives to combat suicide.

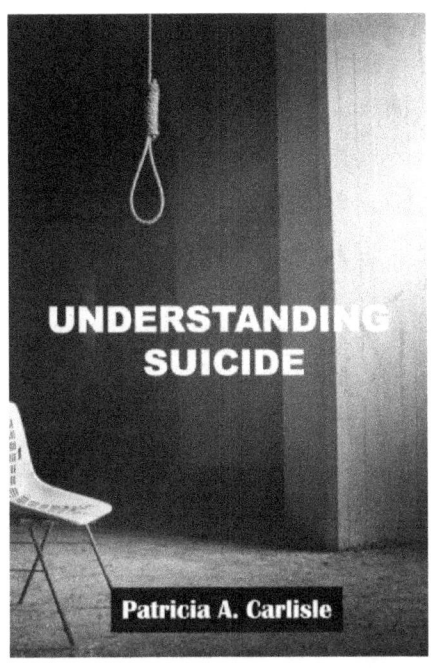

TO CHECK OUT THE REST OF UNDERSTANDING
SUICIDE GO TO AMAZON.COM

Check Out My Other Books

Below you'll find some of my other popular books that are popular on Amazon and Kindle as well. Alternatively, you can visit my author page on Amazon to see other work done by me.

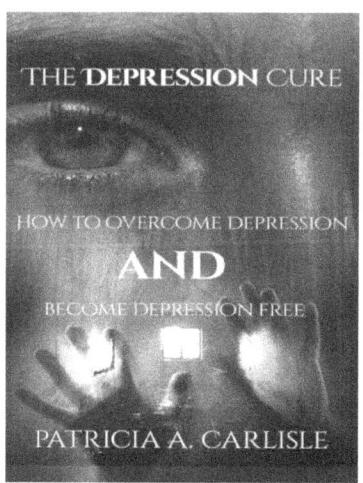

THE DEPRESSION CURE: How to overcome depression and become depression free.

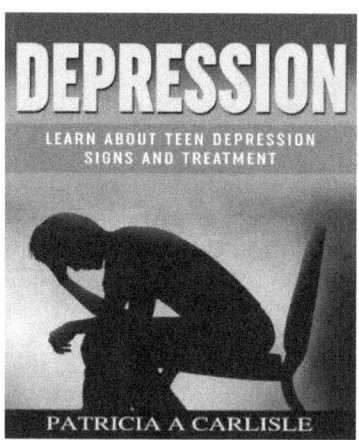

DEPRESSION: Learn About Teen Depression Signs and Treatment.

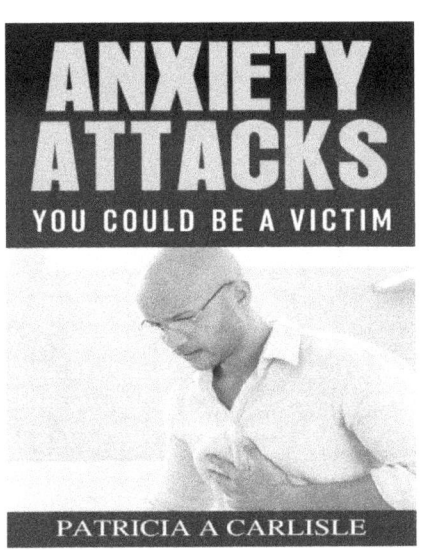

ANXIETY ATTACKS: YOU COULD BE A VICTIM.

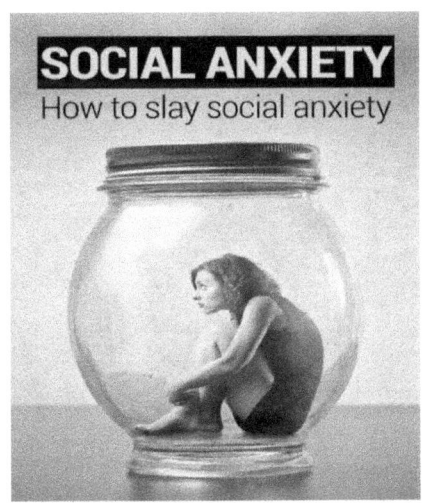

SOCIAL ANXIETY: How to Slay Social Anxiety.

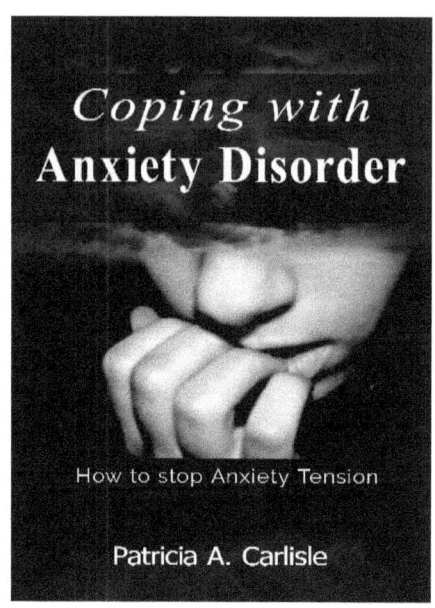

Coping with Anxiety Disorder: How to stop Anxiety Tension.

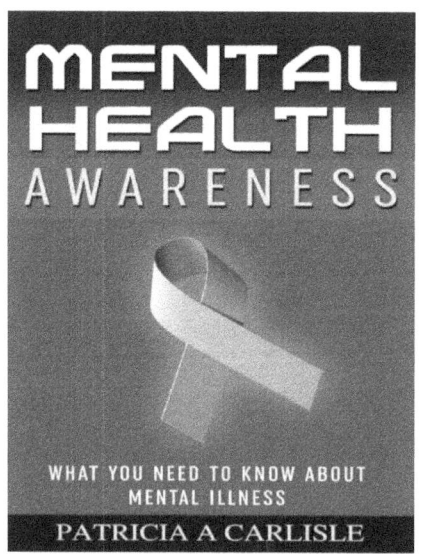

MENTAL HEALTH AWARENESS: What You Need to Know about Mental Illness.

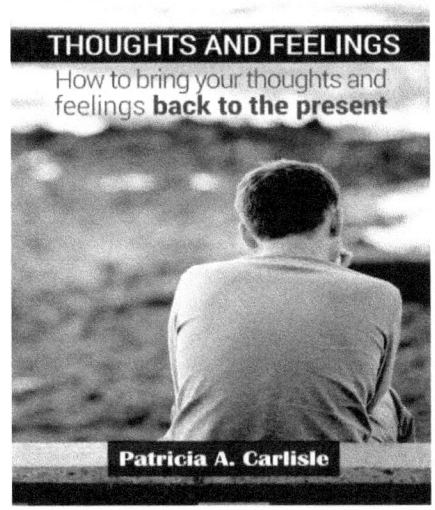

THOUGHTS AND FEELINGS: How to Bring Your Thoughts and Feelings Back to the Present.

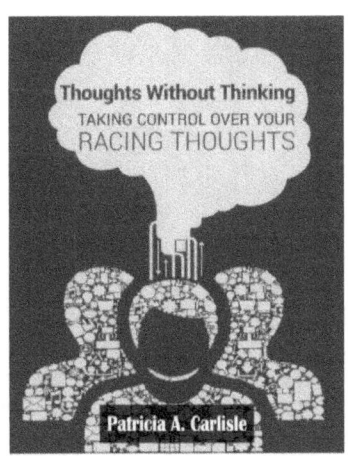

Thoughts Without Thinking: Taking control over your racing thoughts.

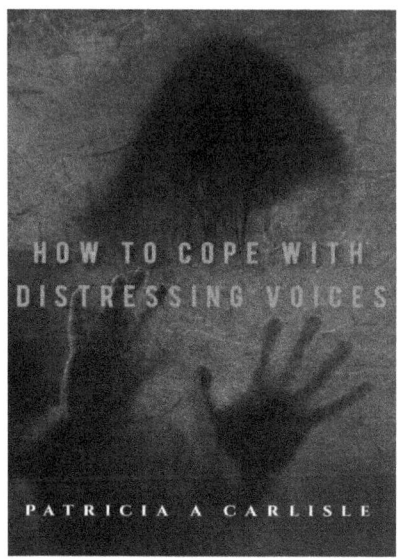

How to cope with distressing voices.

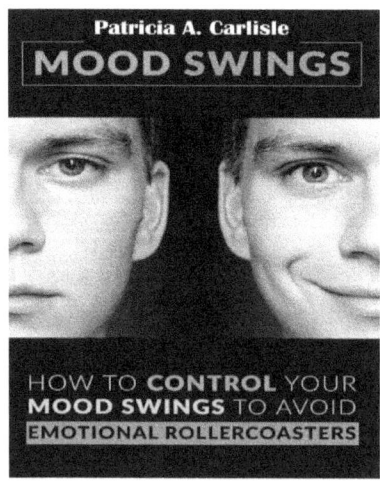

Mood Swings: How to control your mood swings to avoid emotional rollercoster's.

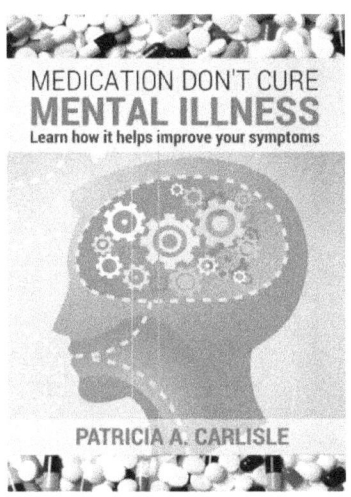

MEDICATION DON'T CURE MENTAL ILLNESS: Learn how it helps improve your symptoms .

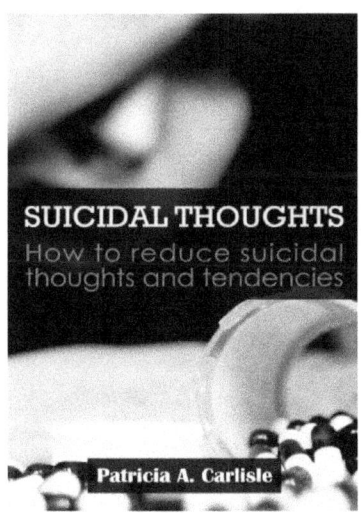

SUICIDAL THOUGHTS: How to Reduce Suicidal Thoughts and Tendencies.

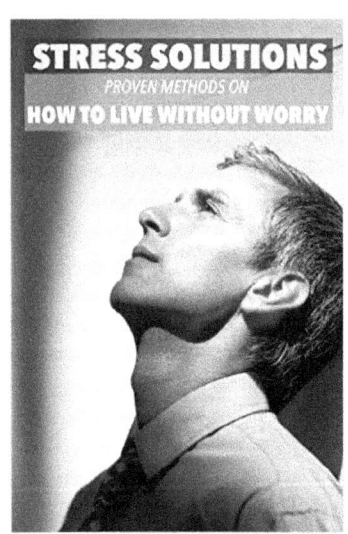

STRESS SOLUTIONS: Proven methods on how to live without worry.

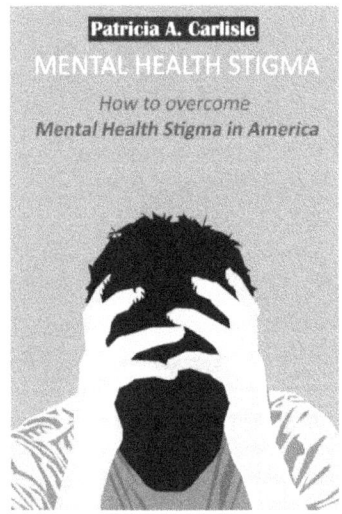

MENTAL HEALTH STIGMA: How to Overcome Mental Health Stigma in America.

BONUS: SUBSCRIBE TO THE FREE BOOK

Beginners Guide to Yoga & Meditation

"Stressed out? Do You Feel Like The World Is Crashing Down Around You? Want To Take A Vacation That Will Relax Your Mind, Body And Spirit? Well this Easy To Read Step By Step

E-Book Makes It All Possible!"

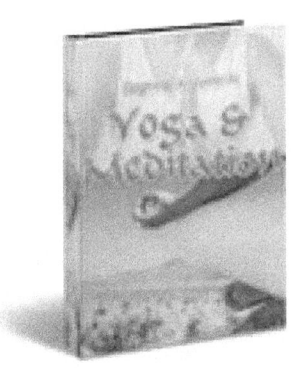

Instructions on how to join our mailing list, and receive a free copy of "Yoga and Meditation" can be found in any of my Kindle eBooks.

NOTES

NOTES

NOTES

NOTES